Maja Bohac
Nikica Gabric
Marija Anticic

Intracor

AF190947

Maja Bohac
Nikica Gabric
Marija Anticic

Intracor

LAP LAMBERT Academic Publishing

Publisher:
LAP LAMBERT Academic Publishing
is a trademark of
Dodo Books Indian Ocean Ltd. and OmniScriptum S.R.L publishing group

120 High Road, East Finchley, London, N2 9ED, United Kingdom
Str. Armeneasca 28/1, office 1, Chisinau MD-2012, Republic of Moldova, Europe
Managing Directors: Ieva Konstantinova, Victoria Ursu
info@omniscriptum.com

Printed at: see last page
ISBN: 978-3-659-30459-0

Contents

1 | Introduction

Marija Anticic MD, Natasa Draca MD

Introduction
Marija Anticic MD, Natasa Draca MD

One of the final frontiers of refractive surgery is the treatment of presbyopia. In the past decades numerous solutions were presented, but the perfect solution is still awaiting to come.

When thinking of presbyopia it is inevitable to come to every individual as the eye ages. Presbyopia is defined as a result of failure of the accommodative mechanism, although precise etiology remains the subject of some debate.

1 Etiology of presbyopia

Understanding the etiology of presbyopia is crucial for the discovery of highly effective methods of its treatment. To bring a nearby object into focus, the ciliary muscle contracts and the tension in the zonules reduces adopting the lens to a thicker and more rounded shape. The deformations that develop in the lens during this process cause the optical power of the eye to increase. In this state the eye is said to be accommodated.[1] As a person ages, the ability to accommodate diminishes, resulting in the condition called presbyopia (Figure 1.1).[2] The most interesting aspect of accommodation is that its time course is well in advance of other physiological functions-it begins to decline by adolescence and is lost about two-thirds of the way through the normal life span. Precise etiology remains the subject of some debate, and many different theories of presbyopia exist. First theory describes presbyopia as a result of crystalline lens hardening.[3]

Second theory describes the lenticular geometric factors, such as an increase in the lens thickness and diameter with age, to be the predominant cause of presbyopia.[2]

Third theory assumes that presbyopia is caused by age related changes in the angle of the zonular attachments to the lens, age related decrease in the ciliary body movement or reduced elasticity of the choroid.[4]

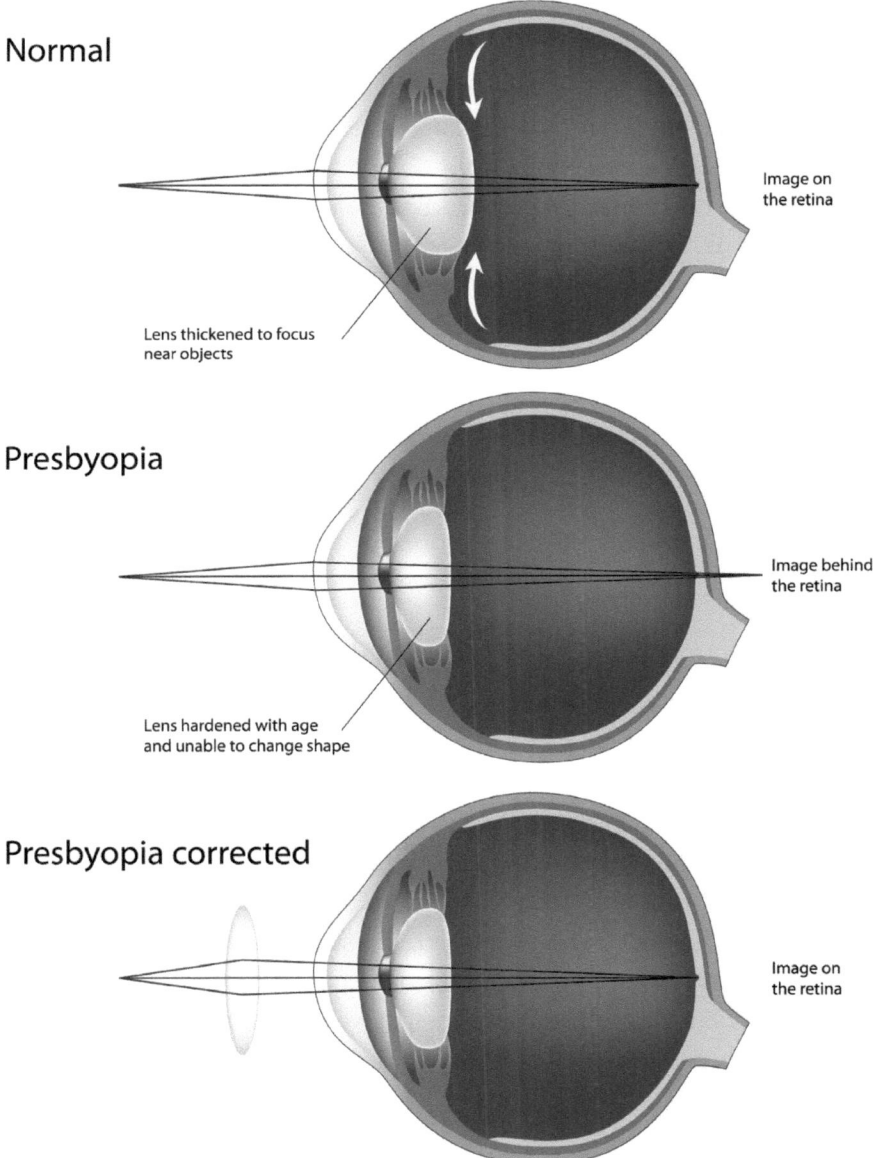

Normal

Image on the retina

Lens thickened to focus near objects

Presbyopia

Image behind the retina

Lens hardened with age and unable to change shape

Presbyopia corrected

Image on the retina

Figure 1.1: Schematic diagram of presbyopia and its effect.

2 Treatment options

Presbyopia can be treated conservatively by prescribing reading glasses and multifocal contact lenses, or with the surgical procedures.

Nowadays, there are numerous surgical techniques which can be accommodative and pseudoaccommodative. Every procedure has limitations and includes some degree of compromise between the distance and near visual acuity outcomes. However, prevalence of presbyopia constantly increases and various correction procedures keep gaining popularity. Accommodative methods for presbyopia treatment comprise implantation of accommodating intraocular lenses (IOLs), scleral expansion procedures and coagulative procedures, while pseudoaccommodative techniques include implantation of multifocal IOLs, corneal inlays, excimer laser-based multifocal ablations and intrastromal femtosecond laser procedures.

2.1 Surgical procedures for treatment of presbyopia

2.1.1 Accommodative procedures

2.1.1.1 Accommodating intraocular lenses (IOLs)

Several designs of accommodating intraocular lenses have been approved for clinical use around the world. Single-optic accommodating IOLs were intended to provide a near visual advantage over monofocal IOLs due to their design, which was claimed to enhance accommodation via an axial lens shift and/or change in lens shape or refractive power. Near visual acuity depends on accommodation and pseudoaccommodation. Some studies of single-optic accommodative IOLs found an advantage of these IOLs over a monofocal IOLs, but unfortunately did not take into a consideration the impact of pseudoaccommodation. So, once pseudoaccommodation was accounted for, there was no advantage in near visual performance with accommodating IOLs over a monofocal IOLs.[5]

Surgical procedures for treatment of presbyopia

Accommodative	Accommodating intraocular lenses (IOLs)
	Scleral expansion procedures
	Coagulative procedures
	Conductive keratoplasty
	YAG laser thermal keratoplasty (LTK)
Pseudoaccommodative	Multifocal IOLs
	Refractive
	Diffractive
	Trifocal
	Corneal inlays
	Excimer laser
	Monovision
	Laser blended vision
	Supracor
	Presbymax
	Femtosecond laser procedures (INTRACOR)

2.1.1.2 Scleral expansion procedures

Schachar introduced a new surgery for presbyopia based on the use of scleral expansion bands (SEB). The aim of these segments was to increase the working distance between the ciliary muscle and the lens equator, which should allow the muscle to work again. The SEB are a development of an initial concept that consisted of a rigid ring increasing the scleral circumference, but this was liable to induce an ischemia of the anterior segment.[6] The modified and improved design of this prototype consists of four polymethylmethacrilate (PMMA) bands that are placed in four scleral tunnels at depths of 350 to 400 micrometers (μm) in order to create more space between the lens and the sclera.[7]

Implantation of the SEB showed high safety for the treatment of presbyopia, while the outcome of the SEB intervention was characterized by inconsistent and unpredictable results with a low level of patient satisfaction.[8]

2.1.1.3 Coagulative procedures

Evolution of thermal techniques to shrink peripheral corneal collagen and thus steepen the central cornea has challenged ophthalmologists for longer than 100 years. Hot-wire thermokeratoplasty, used in the 1980s to produce thermal burns that penetrated to 95% of corneal depth in hyperopic eyes, showed a lack of predictability and stability, and further development was abandoned.[9]

The most current techniques for presbyopia treatment are conductive keratoplasty and yttrium–aluminium–garnet laser thermal keratoplasty (LTK).

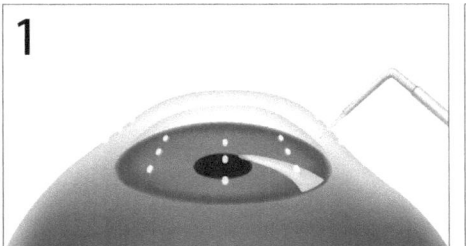 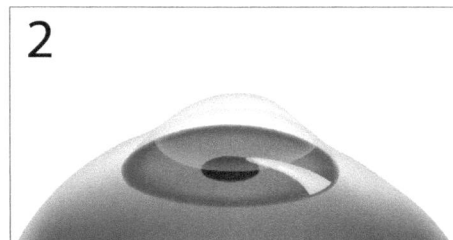

Figure 1.2: Conductive Keratoplasty.

2.1.1.3.1 Conductive keratoplasty

Conductive keratoplasty (CK) is nonablative, radiofrequency-based, collagen-shrinking procedure for the correction of mild to moderate spherical hyperopia for people over the age of 40. Because corneal steepening can add power to the cornea and improve near vision, CK is evaluated for the treatment of presbyopia in emmetropic and hyperopic patients.[10]

Conductive keratoplasty is an electrical current-based technique for shrinking stromal collagen that was originally developed by Mendez et al.[11] It delivers low energy, high frequency (radio frequency, 350 kHz) current directly into the corneal stroma by means of a Keratoplast tip (Refractec, Inc., Irvine, CA) inserted at 16 or more treatment points in the micperipheral cornea *(Figure 1.2)*.[12] Striae form between the treated spots, creating a band of tightening that increases the curvature of the central cornea, thereby decreasing hyperopia.[13]

2.1.1.3.2 YAG laser thermal keratoplasty

YAG laser thermal keratoplasty (LTK) is a procedure that uses laser energy to heat the cornea and increase its curvature. Several reports on the clinical outcome, with the usage of contact LTK devices for the treatment of hyperopia, revealed regression, poor predictability, and significant induced astigmatism.[14]

It was promising in the 1990s, but after the longer follow-up and proven inconsistency of results the procedure was abandoned. [15]

2.1.2 Pseudoaccommodative procedures

2.1.2.1 Multifocal intraocular lenses

Multifocal intraocular lenses (MFIOLs) are designed to provide for distance and near vision without any additional correction. First MFIOLs were introduced in the late 1980s. Those IOLs were designed to provide 2 or more fixed optical powers. Refractive, diffractive and combinations of both optical principles have been developed later. Multifocal intraocular lenses are mostly implanted in cataract patients or in conjunction with clear lens extraction *(Figure 1.3)*.

2.1.2.1.1 Refractive intraocular lenses

The refraction is based on a change in direction of the light ray due to a change in the optical density of the material transmitting the light ray.

The refractive multifocal IOL (ReZOOM, Abbot Medical Optic, USA) has five concentric refractive zones alternating for distance and near vision, with aspheric transitions that allow intermediate vision. Zones 2 and 4 are near dominant and provide +3.5D near addition power at the IOL plane and +2.75D at the spectacle plane (i.e. near point of approximately 39 cm). The distribution of light with this refractive lens is dependent on pupil size. With a 2-mm pupil, approximately 83% of light is directed to the distance focus and 17% to the intermediate focus; with a 5-mm pupil, approximately 60% of light is directed to

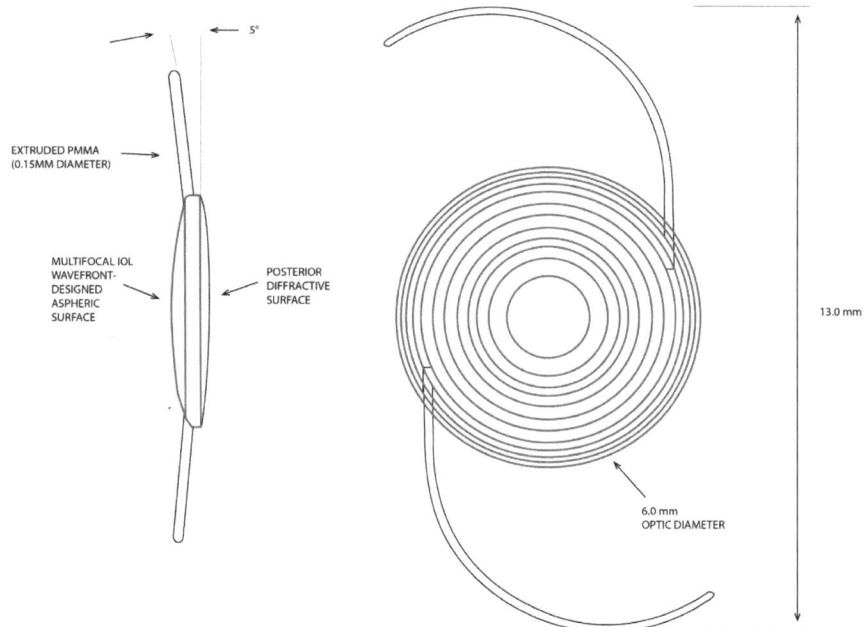

Figure 1.3: Multifocal intraocular lens design.

the distance focus, 30% is directed to the near focus, and 10% is directed to the intermediate focus.[16]

Other example of refractive MFIOLs are Rayner M-flex (Rayner, UK) which provide a degree of pseudoaccommodation, lessening the need for additional refractive correction by spectacles or contact lenses. Those IOLs are based on a multi-zoned refractive aspheric optic technology, with either 4 or 5 annular zones (depending on IOL base power) providing +3.0D or +4.0D of additional refractive power at the IOL plane (equivalent to +2.25D or +3.0D at the spectacle plane).

2.1.2.1.2 Diffractive intraocular lenses

The diffraction is based on the observation that light when encounters a discontinuity or edge in the material in which it travels, scatters in numerous directions.

The AcrySof ReSTOR® IOL (Alcon Laboratories, Inc., Fort Worth, TX) was the first diffractive lens on the market. It uses three optical principles: refraction, diffraction and apodization. Refraction is supposed to enable distance vision and optimize night vision when pupil dilates under scotopic conditions. Diffraction is supposed to provide for distance and near vision in moderate to bright light. Apodization is a gradual reduction or blending of the diffractive step heights which is supposed to improve the efficiency of near vision quality and reduce problems with glare and halos.

The available near addition powers of +2,50, −3,00 and +4,00 diopters provide surgeons the ability to select a treatment option with either a shorter (+4,00D-33 cm) or longer (+3,00D-40 cm and +2,5D-70 cm) reading distance, depending on patient's lifestyle and personal preference. With a 2-mm pupil, this lens design distributes approximately 40% of light for near and 40% for distance, and 20% is lost to higher diffraction orders; for a 5-mm pupil, 84% of light is distributed at distance and 10% for near, and 6% is lost.

Technis IOL (Abbott Medical Optics, USA) is another example of diffractive IOL with reduced spherical aberrations, improved functional vision under low light conditions as well as improved night driving vision.

Acri.LISA multifocal IOL (Carl Zeiss Meditec AG, Jena, Germany) has refractive-diffractive hybrid design features with asymmetric light distribution—65% for distance and 35% for near in both eyes, which is supposed to help in decrease of halos and glare, improve intermediate vision, and provide good distance and near vision under different lighting conditions.

2.1.2.1.3 Trifocal intraocular lenses

These lenses are designed as aspheric multifocal IOLs. Light is distributed asymmetrically through the lens and is independent from the pupil size. Lens design with aberration correcting aspheric optic should reduce light scattering, provide for better contrast sensitivity, depth of field and shaper vision. This design improved intermediate vision and to some extent reduced halos and glare. The latest refractive-diffractive profile design of trifocal lenses provides asymmetrical light distribution of 50%, 20% and 30% for far, intermediate and near which should enable more satisfying and predictable visual outcomes for younger patients with active pupils at all distances (AT LISA tri 839 MP, Carl Zeiss Meditec, Germany). The optical zone of the AT LISA has +3.33D near addition and a +1.66D intermediate addition providing patients with better intermediate vision. Other trifocal lens nowadays on the market are FineVision IOLs Micro F (PhysIOL France), which combine two diffractive structures that are adjusted to offer the +3.5D addition for near vision and +1.75D addition for the intermediate vision.

Side effects. Dissatisfaction after implantation of multifocal IOLs is rare and is usually a consequence of phenomena inherent to the design of multifocal IOL (such as glare and halos), induced astigmatism and poor patient selection.[17]

Careful selection of candidates for multifocal IOLs is mandatory in order to achieve patient's satisfaction. All patients should be educated about what to expect from their vision after surgery. They must be informed about glare and halos immediately following the procedure and the fact that it will get better with time because vision with MFIOLs requires some neuroadaptation. Surgeon should not over-promise the quality of near vision postoperatively, because some patients will still need reading glasses in certain situations. Each lens has its advantages and disadvantages. Refractive lenses give satisfactory far and intermediate vision, while for near tasks additional correction with spectacles is often needed. Diffractive MFIOLs enable satisfactory near and far vision and have no restriction on pupil size, but intermediate vision is poor. The main disadvantage of all multifocal lenses is reduced contrast sensitivity caused by redistribution of light entering an eye to different focal points, and night vision disturbances such as halo and glare.

2.1.2.2 Corneal inlays

Corneal inlays are optical devices inserted into the cornea to reshape the front surface of the eye aiming to improve near and intermediate vision. The main advantage of corneal inlays is the fact that there is no tissue removal and that they can be removed if necessary.

Corneal inlays are usually implanted in the nondominant eye using flaps or pockets created by microkeratome or femtosecond laser. The inlays are usually very small with 2-4mm of overall diameter and 15-20μm of thickness. They are placed on the corneal bed and usually centered on the pupil.

There are several types of corneal inlays on the market. Kamra Inlay (AcuFocus, Inc., Irvine, California, USA) has small–aperture optics which increases the depth of field.[18] Raindrop Near vision inlay (ReVision Optics, Lake Forest, California, USA) has the same refractive index as cornea and is intended only to increase the curvature of central cornea resulting in more prolate shape.[19]

Flexivue Micro-Lens (Presbia, Los Angeles, California, USA) is designed to change the eye's refractive index. It has bifocal design with plano central zone and peripheral rings of varying addition power for near vision.[20]

Recent studies showed average increase of 5 or more lines of uncorrected near visual acuity after the implantation of corneal inlays. However, all inlays showed significant decrease in uncorrected distance visual acuity and loss of lines of best corrected distance visual acuity in the operated eye. Also, there are some reports about increase of high order aberrations, decrease in contrast sensitivity and night vision problems after the implantation of corneal inlays.

Longer follow up and larger series of patients are needed to demonstrate safety and efficaccy of this promising surgical method.

2.1.2.3 Excimer laser

2.1.2.3.1 Monovision

In monovision surgery the patient has 1 eye (usually non dominant) corrected for near tasks, and the other eye (dominant) corrected for distance vision. Patients who are dissatisfied with monovision have strong sighting preferences, significant reduction in stereo acuity, minimal interocular blur suppression and large esophoric shifts with monovision.[21]

Success depends on interocular suppression of blur. Presbyopia correction by using LASIK is attractive because it is a well-established surgical technique and offers the ability of easy enhancement.

2.1.2.3.1.1 Laser blended vision (Carl Zeiss Meditec)

Laser Blended Vision is different from traditional monovision because it increases the depth of field of each eye. Depth of field in this procedure is drawn on 5 mechanisms: (1) a specific controlled increase in corneal spherical aberration, (2) pupil constriction during accommodation affording further depth of field increase on the retinal image, (3) retinal and cortical processing for increasing contrast of the retinal image monocularly, (4) blend zone to enable continuous distance to intermediate to near vision between the two eyes and (5) central cortical processing including neuronal gating and blur-suppression.[22]

Laser Blended Vision is a treatment option for presbyopia correction in patients with emmetropia, myopia and hyperopia, even in the presence of astigmatism. It can be used to treat refractive errors between +5.75 and -9.00D.

Laser Blended Vision combines nonlinear aspheric ablation profiles with micro-monovision.

2.1.2.3.2 Supracor (Technolas Perfect Vision GmbH)

Supracor is a new-generation excimer laser pseudoaccommodative corne-al treatment that can simultaneously treat patients' distance and near correc-tion. It uses a progressive ablation profile to provide an aberration-optimized smooth transition from distance to near correction.[23]

The Supracor algorithm performs a central ablation (INTRACOR-like) for near vision (central 3.00 mm zone with emmetropia as a target for both eyes) and a paracentral ablation for distance vision (multifocal corneal profile over a 6.0 mm optical zone).[24] A disadvantage of these procedure is loss of lines of CDVA which is potential drawback of many presbyopia procedures and also reduced UDVA in some eyes due to overcorrection toward greater degrees of myopia than intended.[23]

2.1.2.3.3 Presbymax (Schwind Eye Tech Solutions)

Presbymax integrates biaspheric multifocal ablation profiles into two focus-shifted aspheric profiles with different asphericities. It uses wavefront diagnostic data as well as presbyopic compensation, thereby combining the advantages of both techniques—improved visual outcomes and enhanced pseudoaccommo-dation. The profile meets the following requirements: multifocality (the center is corrected for near and the periphery for far vision), optimized biaspheric profile, and addition of a precalculated amount of higher-order spherical aberrations.

2.1.2.4 Femtosecond laser procedures (INTRACOR)

INTRACOR is a femtosecond laser procedure designed to improve near vision by making intrastromal corneal cuts, leading to a multifocal cornea and increasing the central corneal steepness while preserving the corneal epithelium *(Figure 1.4)*. Therefore, it is minimally invasive with a minimum risk for infection.[25]

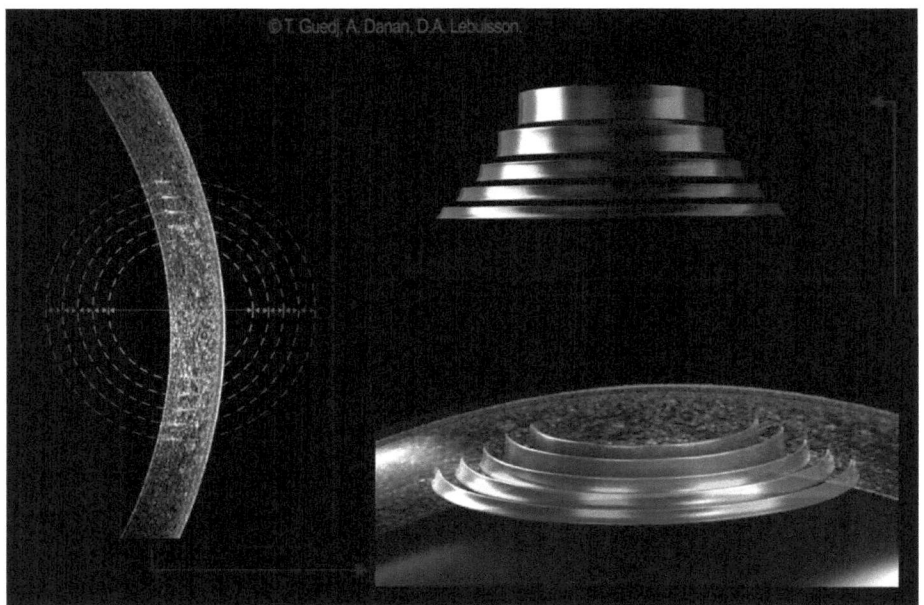

Figure 1.4: INTRACOR- intrastromal corneal cuts, leading to a multifocal cornea.

References:

1. Burd HJ, Wilde GS, Judge SJ. An improved spinning lens test to determine the stiffness of the human lens. Exp Eye Res 2011;92(1):28-39.

2. Strenk SA, Strenk LM, Koretz JF. The mechanism of presbyopia. Progress in Retina and Eye Research 2005;24:379–393.

3. Heys KR, Cram SL, Truscott RJ. Massive increase in the stiffness of the human lens nucleus with age: the basis for presbyopia? Mol Vision 2004;10:956–963.

4. Wyatt HJ. Application of a simple mechanical model of accommodation to the aging eye. Vision Research 1993;33:731–738.

5. Beiko GHH. Comparison of visual results with accommodating intraocular lenses versus mini-monovision with a monofocal intraocular lens. J Cataract Refract Surg 2013;39:48-55.

6. Malecaze FJ, Gazagne CS, Tarroux MC, et al. Scleral expansion bands for presbyopia. Ophtalmology 2001;108(12):2165-2171.

7. Holzer MP, Sandoval H, Solomon KD. Surgery for Presbyopia. AAO, Refractive Management vol 1: Module 3.

8. Qazi MA, Pepose JS, Shuster JJ. Implantation of scleral expansion band segments for the treatment of presbyopia. Am J Ophtalmol 2002;134:808-815.

9. McDonald MB, Hersh PS, Manche EE et al. Conductive keratoplasty for the correction of low to moderate hyperopia U.S. Clinical trial 1-year results on 355 eyes. Ophtalmology 2002;109(11):1978-1989.

10. McDonald MB, Durrie D, Asbell P, et al. Treatment of presbyopia with conductive keratoplasty, six-month results of the 1-year United States FDA clinical trial. Cornea 2004;23(7):661-669.

11. Mendez A, Mendez Noble A. Conductive keratoplasty for the correction of hyperopia. In: Sher NA, ed. Surgery for Hyperopia and Presbyopia. Baltimore: Lippincott Williams & Wilkins;1997:163–171

12. Goth P, Stern R. Conductive keratoplasty: Principles and technology. Presented at a meeting of the American Society for Cataract and Refractive Surgery, April 2000 Boston.

13. McDonald MB, Davidorf J, Maloney RK, et al. Conductive keratoplasty for the correction of low to moderate hyperopia. Ophtalmology 2002;109(4):637-649.

14. Tutton MK, Cherry PM. Holmium: YAG laser thermokeratoplasty to correct hyperopia: two years follow-up. Ophthalmic Surg Lasers 1996;27(5):521–524.

15. Koch DD, Kohnen T, McDonnell PJ, et al. Hyperopia correction by noncontact holmium: YAG laser thermal keratoplasty. U.S. phase IIA clinical study with 2-year follow-up. Ophthalmology 1997;104(11):1938–1947.

16. Chiam PJ, Chan JH, Aggarwal RK, et al. ReSTOR intraocular lens implantation in cataract surgery: quality of vision. J Cataract Refract Surg 2006;32(9):149–163.

17. Dexl AK, Seyeddain O, Riha W, et al. Reading performance after implantation of a modified corneal inlay design for the surgical correction of presbyopia: 1-year follow-up. Am J Ophtalmol 2012;153(5):994-1001.

18. Seyeddain O, Hohensinn M, Riha W, et al. Small-aperture corneal inlay for the correction of presbyopia: 3-year follow-up. J Cataract Refract Surg 2012;38(1):35-45.

19. Porter T, Lang A, Holliday K, et al. Clinical performance of a hydrogel corneal inlay in hyperopic presbyopes. Invest Vis Ophth Sci 2012; 53: abstract 4056.

20. Limnopoulou AN, Bouzoukis DI, Kymionis GD, et al. Visual outcomes and safety of a refractive corneal inlay for presbyopia using femtosecond laser. J Refract Surg 2013;29(1):12-18.

21. Ryan A, O'Keefe M. Corneal approach to hyperopic presbyopia treatment: six-month outcomes of a new multifocal excimer laser in situ keratomileusis

procedure. J Cataract Refract Surg 2013;39(8):1226-1233.

22. Reinstein DZ, Archer TJ, Gobbe M. Aspheric ablation profile for presbyopic corneal treatment using the MEL80 and CRS Master Laser Blended Vision module. J Emmetropia 2011;2:161-175.

23. Soler Tomás JR, Fuentes-Páez G, Burillo S. Asymmetrical Supracor for hyperopic presbyopes: short term results. J Emmetropia 2013; 4:79-85.

24. Evans BJ. Monovision: a review. Ophthalmic Physiol Opt 2007;27(5):417-439.

25. Menassa N, Fitting A, Auffarth GU, et al. Visual outcomes and corneal changes after intrastromal femtosecond laser correction of presbyopia. J Cataract Refract Surg 2012;38:765–773.

2 Intrastromal correction of presbyopia (INTRACOR)

Maja Bohac MD,
Marija Anticic MD

Intrastromal correction of presbyopia (INTRACOR)

Maja Bohac MD, Marija Anticic MD

After the feasibility of the intracorneal correction has been shown by numerous studies, the first patients were treated in October 2007 by the Columbian surgeon and innovator in the field of refractive surgery Dr Luis Ruiz.

He initially treated emmetropic presbyopic patients with the TECHNOLAS femtosecond laser and later also patients with other refractive errors such as myopia, hyperopia and/or astigmatism. He presented his results for the first time at the Royal Hawaiian Meeting in January 2008 and attracted a lot of attention among the present experts.

In order to further study and develop this new procedure named INTRACOR, a multicentre Conformite Europeenne (CE) study was started in four sites in Germany in the same year. The surgeons from the clinics and hospitals involved in the study were Priv.-Doz. Dr. Mike Holzer and Prof. Dr. Gerd Auffarth from Heidelberg as well as Dr. Mark Tomalla from Duisburg, Prof. Dr. Michael Knorz from Mannheim and Dr. Tobias Neuhann from Munich. The positive outcome of the study resulted in the procedure for presbyopic patients with minor degrees of hyperopia, obtaining CE approval in April 2009.

1 CE approval study for INTRACOR

After the approval from the Ethics Committee of Ruprecht-Karls University of Heidelberg, patients were recruited for the prospective multicentre study in four sites in Germany (Duisburg, Heidelberg, Mannheim and Munich) from June 2008 onwards. The first treatments took place in July 2008 and by October 2008 a total of 63 patients had been included and treated in the study. After providing detailed patient information and written consent to participate in the study, the patients were consecutively enrolled at the individual study sites until the number of patients needed for the statistical evaluation calculated beforehand (n=63) had been reached. All patients treated in the study were allowed to have treatment on one eye, which was the non-dominant eye. All treatments were performed without any complications by the investigators in the presence of an application specialist from the Technolas Perfect Vision at each study site. The mean age of the patients was 55±6.2 years (range 43 to 72 years); of the 63 patients 23 were women (36.5%) and 40 men (63.5%). The inclusion criteria was that, besides presbyopia with a required near vision addition of +2.00 diopter (D) or more, the patients also had to have distance refraction between +0.5 to +1.25D. The cylinder had to be maximum of 0.5D and the spherical equivalent (SE) between +0.25 and +1.00D. Patients were not allowed to have any other eye disease or previous surgery. The surgery and postoperative regimen were conducted according to the Technolas general recommendations.

The mean preoperative uncorrected distance visual acuity was 0.13±0.11 logMAR, and near visual acuity was 0.72±0.17 logMAR. Preoperative spherical refraction was +0.74±0.37D and cylinder was 0.29±0.4D.

Postoperatively, there was almost no change in the mean uncorrected distance visual acuity and at six months follow up it was 0.11±0.12 logMAR. There was a significant increase in the uncorrected near visual acuity. On the near vision chart used, at the distance of 40cm the gain was 4.6±2.0 lines, which was equivalent to a logMAR near vision of 0.26±0.19. Postoperative spherical refraction decreased to a mean of 0.56±0.44D, while there was almost no change in cylinder.

Improvements in uncorrected distance visual acuity and decrease in spherical correction were explained by the fact that a minimal myopic shift was achieved through INTRACOR treatment for presbyopia. Patients who preoperatively had minor hyperopia came closer to being almost emmetropic.

Topography measurements showed central steepening of the cornea and somewhat more pronounced negative asphericity of the cornea.

During the follow up period there were no severe adverse or undesirable effects observed, and the achieved visual acuities remained stable.

References:

1. Holzer MP, Mannsfeld A, Ehmer A, Auffarth GU. Early outcomes of IN-TRACOR femtosecond laser treatment for presbyopia. J Refract Surg. 2009;25:855-861.

2. Ruiz LA, Cepeda LM, Fuentes VC. Intrastromal correction of presbyopia using a femtosecond laser system. J Refract Surg.2009;25:847-854

3. Tomalla M. Femtosecond Laser-Principles and Application in Ophthalmology. 1st ed. Bremen:UNI-MED,2010:82-86.

4. Holzer MP, Knorz MC, Tomalla M, Neuhann TM, Auffarth GU. Intrastromal femtosecond laser presbyopia correction: 1-year results of a multicenter study. J Refract Surg. 2012;28(3):182-188.

5. Ruiz LA. Preliminary clinical results with 12-months follow-up of intrastromal correction of presbyopia using the FEMTEC femtosecond laser system and INTRACOR procedure. Data provided by the 20/10 Perfect Vision, Heidelberg, Germany.

3 INTRACOR principle of work

**Maja Bohac MD,
Nikica Gabric MD, PhD**

INTRACOR principle of work

Maja Bohac MD, Nikica Gabric MD, PhD

By using the femtosecond laser a customized pattern is applied into the cornea inducing a local reorganization of the biomechanical forces *(Figure 3.1)*. In presbyopia treatment the applied pattern leads to a locally well-defined central steepening of the cornea, resulting in the central increase of refractive power. As the refractive power change is only centrally induced, a significant increase of near vision is evoked whereas the distance vision is only minimally affected. The femtosecond laser by means of local photodisruption of tissue creates five cylindrical ring incisions of different heights inside the cornea, starting above Descemet's membrane and ending approximately 100µm below Bowman's membrane *(Figure 3.2)*. The innermost cylinder is 1.8mm in the CE-certified version *(Figure 3.3 and Figure 3.4)*.

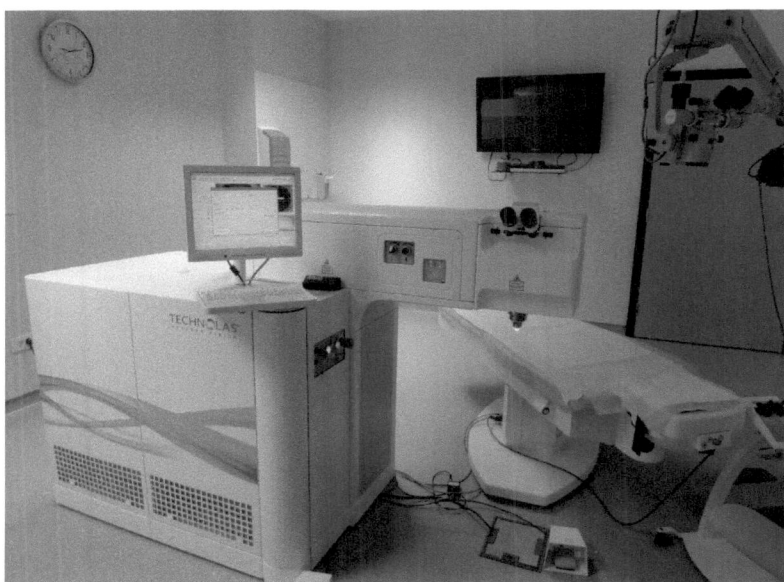

Figure 3.1: TECHNOLAS® Femtosecond 520F Workstation.

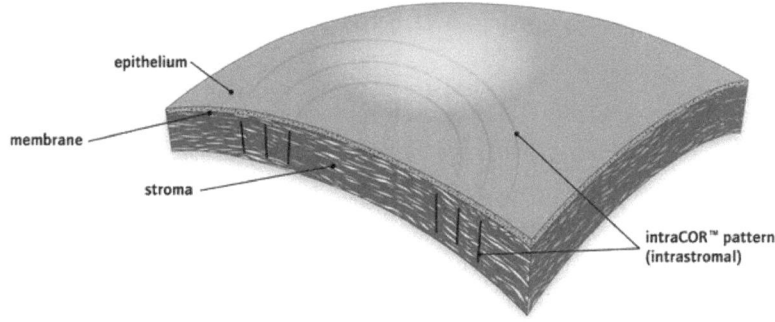

Figure 3.2: Diagram of the five intrastromal rings which lead to slight steepening of the central cornea.

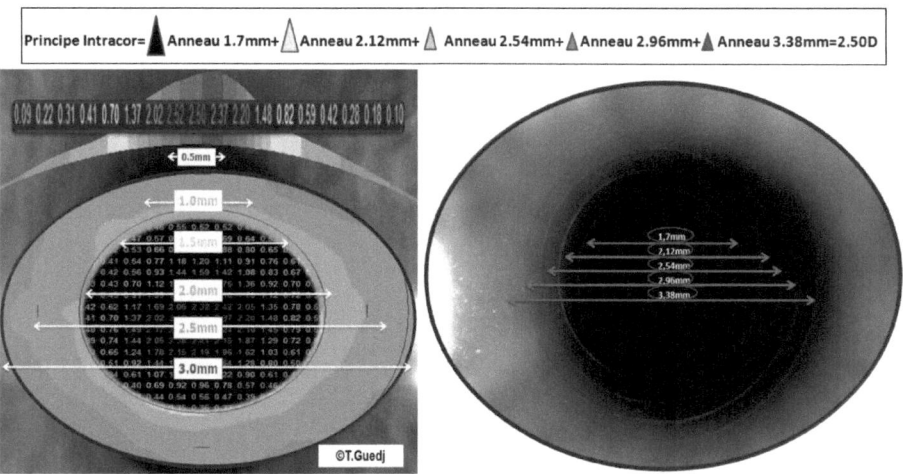

Figure 3.3: Diagram of INTRACOR cylinder width.

The principle of INTRACOR is that the intraocular pressure pushes the innermost part of the cornea slightly forward, to create a small change in position (5-8µm), and results in central steepening of the cornea without inducing any change to the periphery and mid-periphery *(Figure 3.5)*. Additionally, there is an induction of negative spherical aberration, which is important because it increases patient's depth of focus and allows them to see better at near. As a small side effect, it also induces approximately -0.50D of myopia. The procedure is astigmatically neutral.

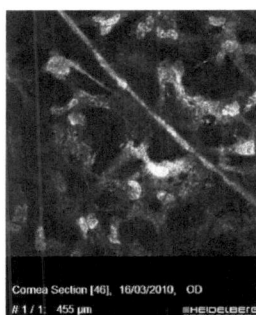

Figure 3.4: Cornea-specific in vivo laser scanning confocal microscope (Heidelberg Retina Tomograph 2 Rostock Cornea Module, HRT2-RCM)-image of intrastromal cut.

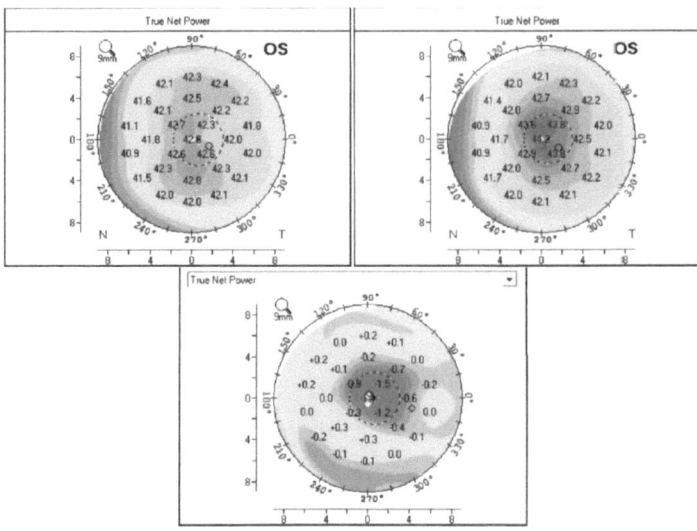

Figure 3.5: Difference in preoperative and postoperative corneal topography with increase in central corneal steepening after the procedure.

27

References:

1. Tomalla M. Femtosecond Laser-Principles and Application in Ophthalmology. 1st ed. Bremen: UNI-MED, 2010:82-86.

2. Holzer MP, Knorz MC, Tomalla M, Neuhann TM, Auffarth GU. Intrastromal femtosecond laser presbyopia correction: 1-year results of a multicenter study. J Refract Surg. 2012; 28(3):182-188.

3. An excerpt from the presentation by Dr Luis Ruiz and Dr Mike Holzer and the roundtable discussion moderated by Dr Wing-Kwong Chan in the 1st Technolas Perfect Vision Aliance. Bali: 15 May 2009.

4. Knorz MC. 12-Month Conformité Europeénne Data on INTRACOR. Supplement to Cataract and Refractive Surgery Today Europe. June 2010: 3-5.

5. Ruiz LA, Cepeda LM, Fuentes VC. Intrastromal correction of presbyopia using a femtosecond laser system. J Refract Surg.2009; 25:847-854.

4 Patient selection for INTRACOR

Maja Bohac MD,
Marija Anticic MD,
Nikica Gabric MD, PhD

Patient selection for INTRACOR

Maja Bohac MD, Marija Anticic MD, Nikica Gabric MD, PhD

As in all refractive patients, thorough and exhaustive preliminary examinations are needed before deciding on whether to undertake INTRACOR treatment of presbyopia.

There is a need to determine the manifest and especially cycloplegic refraction to rule out any latent hyperopia. Ideal patient should have at least +1.50D for near addition. Refraction for distance should not exceed +1.0D in spherical equivalent. Cylinder should not be more than 0.5D.

Slit lamp and dilated fundus examination should be performed. Patients with cataract and any form of evolutive retinal pathology, especially macular pathology, should be excluded.

Corneal topography is mandatory diagnostic method that needs to be evaluated. Cornea should be at least 500µm thick in the thinnest point. Minimum keratometry readings should be at least 40.0D, while maximum keratometry readings should not exceed 48.8D. Difference between minimum and maximum keratometry readings should not be more than 2.0D. *(Figure 4.1)*.

Pupilography should be performed, and all patients with > 6.5mm pupil in scotopic condition should be excluded.

Patients with any sign of corneal dystrophy, especially ectatic disorders, should be ruled out.

Since the exact effect on measurement of the intraocular pressure has not yet been definitely investigated, glaucoma patients should also not be treated.

The non-dominant eye should be treated first. It is recommended to perform contact lens trial preoperatively to test patient's acceptance of potential decrease in the distance vision. The INTRACOR eye should be set to a refraction of -0.50D. However, we have to have in mind that monovision is not the target of the treatment because INTRACOR aims for near and distance correction.

Dominant eye can be treated after at least 4 weeks and only in patients who specially request treatment of the other eye and if no significant loss in distance visual acuity in the operated eye was observed.

INTRACOR treatment after excimer laser surgery is conceivable and has already been undertaken in individual cases but was not reviewed within the scope of the CE study. Furthermore the biomechanical response of the corneal tissue is currently more difficult to predict. There are some post cataract cases which received INTRACOR with very promising results, and that is a viable option for patients who received monofocal IOL seeking for presbyopia solution.

The most important part in selection of patients is preoperative chair time. It is crucial for patients to understand that INTRACOR does not make their presbyopia disappear but rather decrease the symptoms of presbyopia. In comparison to multifocal intraocular lenses patients will have to have some reading glasses for small print and low light conditions. However, they will undergo less invasive surgery without potential intraocular complications and night vision disturbances that clear lens extraction with multifocal IOL implantation can produce.

OCULUS - PENTACAM

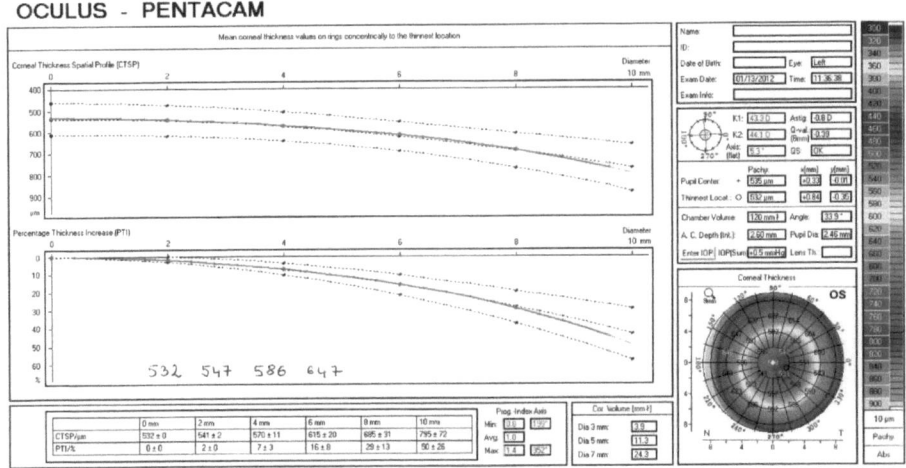

Figure 4.1: Corneal topography (Pentacam High Resolution; Oculus, Wetzlar, Germany).

References:

1. Holzer MP, Knorz MC, Tomalla M, Neuhann TM, Auffarth GU. Intrastromal femtosecond laser presbyopia correction: 1-year results of a multicenter study. J Refract Surg. 2012;28:182-188.

2. Ruiz LA, Cepeda LM, Fuentes VC. Intrastromal correction of presbyopia using a femtosecond laser system. J Refract Surg. 2009;25:847-854.

3. Tomalla M. Femtosecond Laser-Principles and Application in Ophthalmology. 1st ed. Bremen: UNI-MED, 2010:82-86.

4. Personal communication with application specialist from Technolas Perfect Vision, Munich, Germany.

5. A CG, Ruiz B, Gomez P, Antelo M. Experience with INTRACOR in Special Presbyopia Cases. Supplement to Cataract and Refractive Surgery Today Europe. June 2010:8-10.

6. Holzer MP, Mannsfeld A, Ehmer A, Auffarth GU. Early outcomes of INTRACOR femtosecond laser treatment for presbyopia. J Refract Surg. 2009; 25:855-861.

5 Surgery and postoperative regimen

**Maja Bohac MD,
Marija Anticic MD,
Nikica Gabric MD, PhD**

Surgery and postoperative regimen
Maja Bohac MD, Marija Anticic MD, Nikica Gabric MD, PhD

Prior to the surgery it is recommended to check the laser parameters, enter the patient's data and pachymetry values *(Figure 5.1 and 5.2)*. Afterwards, specific curved patient's interface is connected to a laser cone and central marking has to be done prior to the patient alignment.

Patient's eye is anaesthetized with oxybuprocaine hydrochloride 0.4% drops prior to the surgery. After positioning the patient on the bed, under the surgical microscope the line of sight is marked with a sharp instrument using the Purkinje image *(Figure 5.3)*.

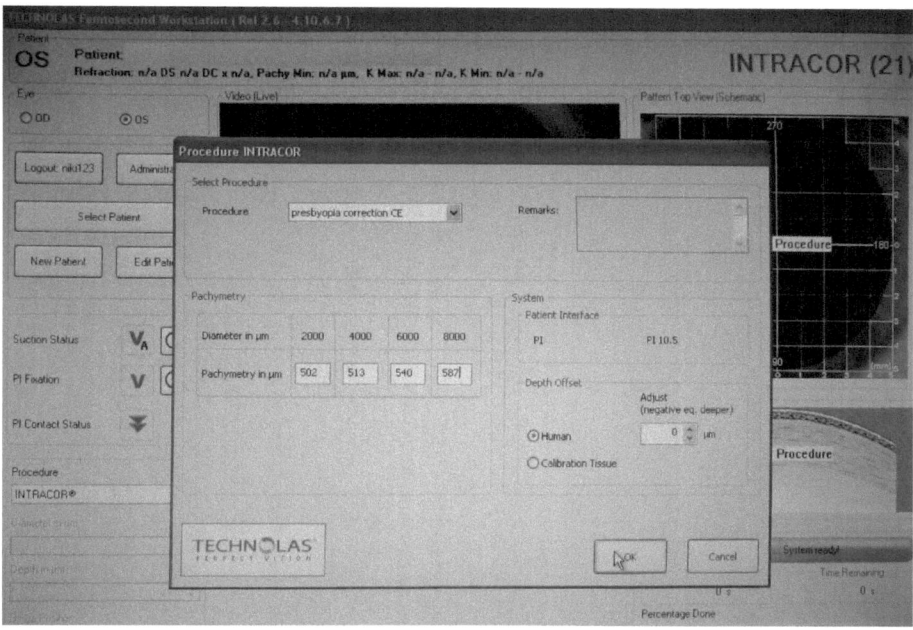

Figure 5.1: Preoperative planning inside the laser.

34

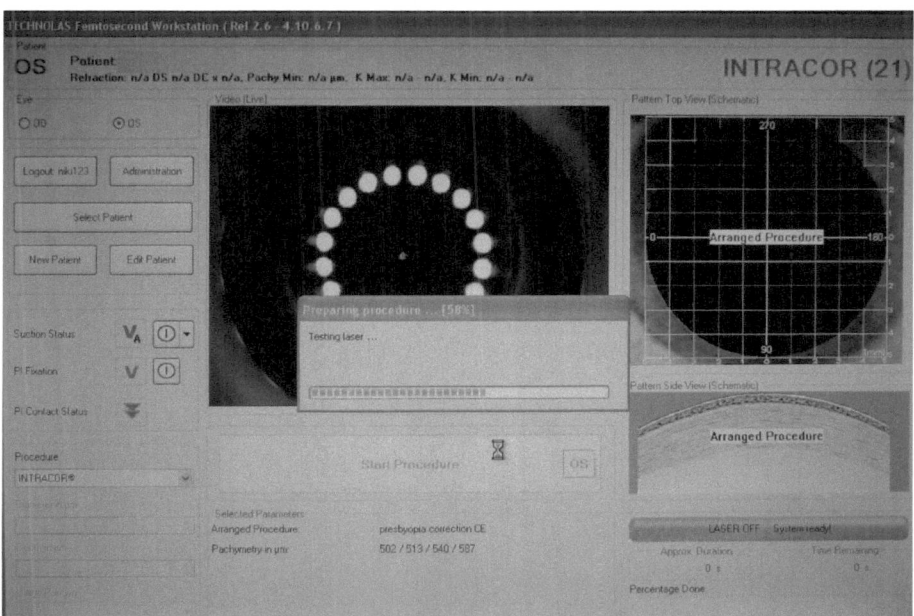

Figure 5.2: Preoperative planning inside the laser.

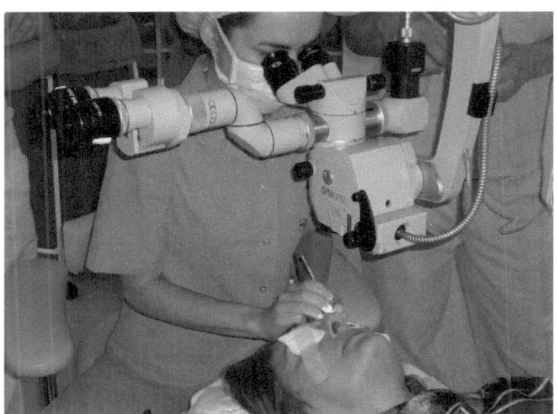

Figure 5.3: The line of sight is marked with a sharp instrument using the Purkinje image under the surgical microscope.

35

Suction ring with the centering cross is placed on the eye. After aligning the center of the cross to the marking, vacuum is applied. When accurate positioning and adequate vacuum level is achieved, the suction ring is opened and centering cross carefully removed. The patient's bed is swiveled under the laser and patient is asked to look at the red fixation light. Precision of manual centering is checked once again since red reflex of the light and the manually created mark should coincide. As the pattern is generated very centrally, it is essential for this procedure to align the pattern very properly on the patient's line of sight to avoid postoperative vision disturbances *(Figure 5.4 and 5.5)*.

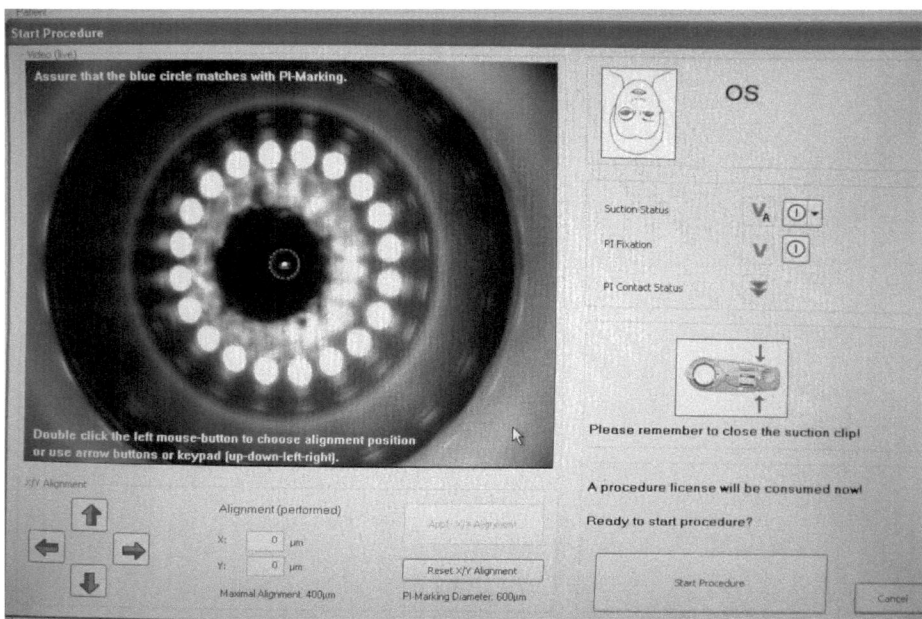

Figure 5.4: Precise manual centering to align the pattern very properly on the patient's line of sight.

The eye is then connected to the femtosecond laser using a specific curved patient's interface device and suction ring is closed.

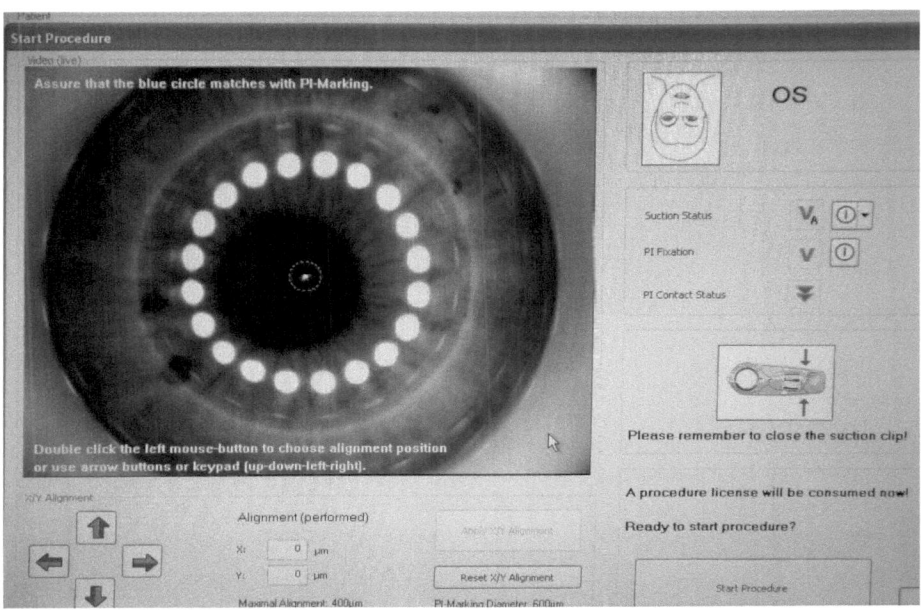

Figure 5.5: Pattern is generated very centrally, red reflex of the light and the manually created mark should coincide.

After appropriate positioning and closing, the laser is applied and five pure-
ly intrastromal consecutive rings around the line of sight are cut with the laser
beam *(Figure 5.6, 5.7 and 5.8)*.

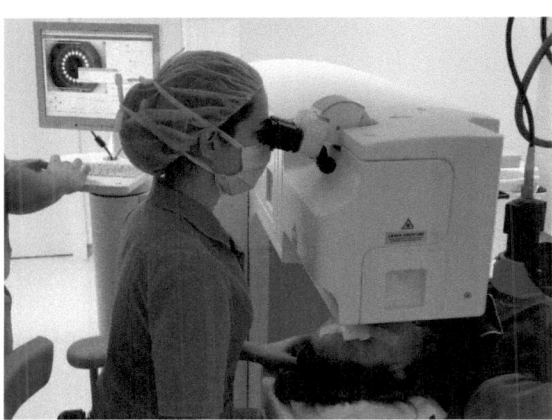

*Figure 5.6: Intervention-
INTRACOR procedure using
the TECHNOLAS® Femto-
second 520F Workstation.*

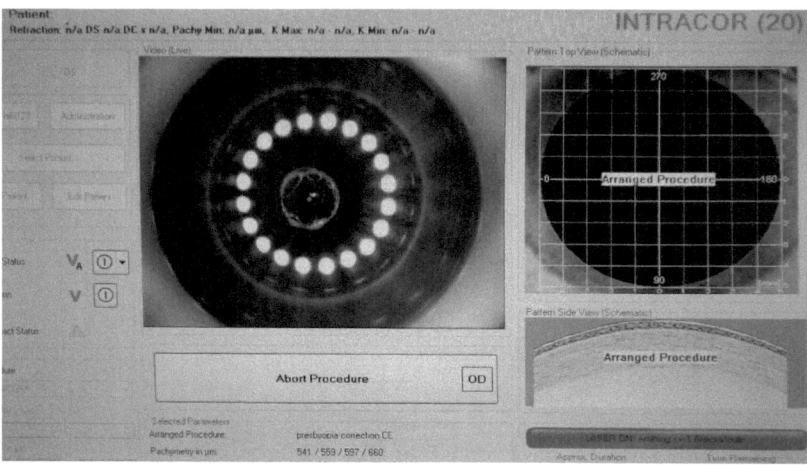

Figure 5.7: Beginning of laser application, first intrastromal ring around the line of sight is cut with the laser beam.

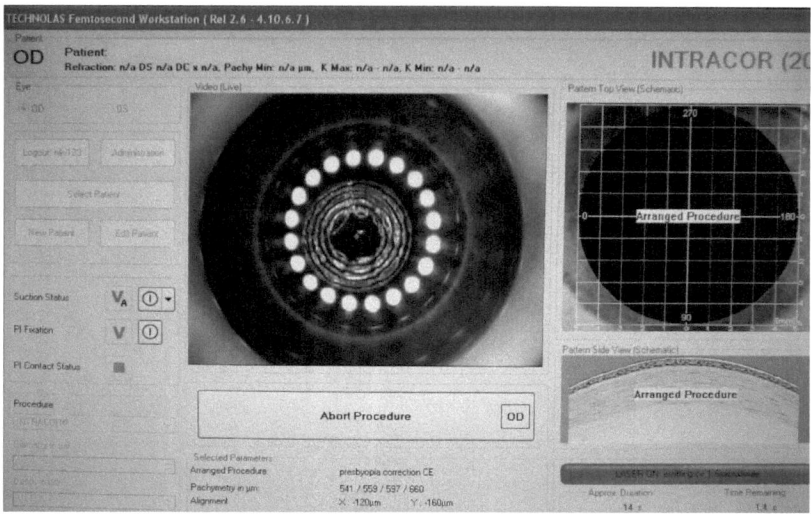

Figure 5.8: Formation of five concentric rings after centration of the patient interface by means of ring illumination and the Purkinje reflex.

38

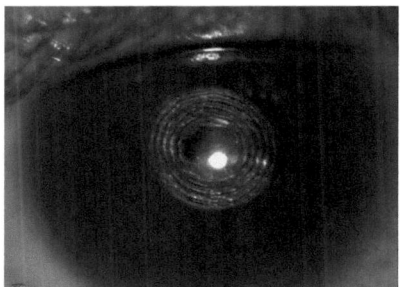

Figure 5.9: Slit lamp findings in a presbyopic eye that was treated with IN-TRACOR. The photograph shows the findings 1 hour postoperatively and ring cuts are still somewhat expanded as a result of gas that arises during tissue photodisruption. The gas escapes during the first two or three hours post-op.

1 Options for retreatment

There is still no available long term study of INTRACOR retreatments. Few options are still in the process of investigation. One of the options include 6th deeper ring, and another one just repeating available 5 ring procedure on top of the previous one. The biggest issue in the repeated procedure is centering.

References:

1. Bohac M, Gabric N, Anticic M, Draca N, Dekaris I. First results of INTRACOR procedure in Croatia. Coll. Antropol. 2011;35(2):161-166.

2. Holzer MP, Mannsfeld A, Ehmer A, Auffarth GU. Early outcomes of IN-TRACOR femtosecond laser treatment for presbyopia. J Refract Surg. 2009; 25:855-861.

3. Personal communication with application specialist from Technolas Perfect Vision, Munich, Germany.

6 Results

**Maja Bohac MD,
Nikica Gabric MD, PhD**

Results
Maja Bohac MD, Nikica Gabric MD, PhD

INTRACOR as a treatment method for presbyopia is used in our clinic since December 2010. Until now more than 400 eyes were treated with this procedure. 71 patients (95 eyes) have completed a two years follow up. In these early days we performed much more binocular treatments than we are doing nowadays. Furthermore, in the first group of patients 23 out of 71 patients received binocular treatment.

The mean age of patients was 54.22±4.22 years (range 46-63 years); of the 72 patients 69% were men and 31% were women. The mean preoperative spherical equivalent (SE) was 0.74±0.29 (range plano to +1.25D). The mean monocular uncorrected distance visual acuity (UDVA) was 0.71±0.21 (range 0.6 to 1.0), while the mean monocular corrected distance visual acuity (CDVA) was 0.98±0.03 (range 0.9 to 1.0). The mean monocular uncorrected near visual acuity (UNVA) was 0.34±0.2 (range J3 to J16), while the mean monocular corrected near visual acuity (CNVA) was 0.95±0.03 (range J1 to J2). The mean binocular UDVA was 0.81±0.19 (range 0.7 to 1.0), while the mean binocular UNVA was 0.39±0.24 (range J3 to J16).

All treatments were performed without any complications. After the standard thorough preoperative examination, the surgery was performed. The procedure and postoperative regimen were applied as previously described. Patients were followed up on day 1 and 7, then after 1, 3 and 6 months, and after 1 and 2 years *(Figure 6.1, 6.2 and 6.3)*. Uncorrected monocular and binocular distance and near visual acuity, and changes in the central corneal power were measured. Statistical analysis was performed using Students t-test with p value ≤0.05 as statistically significant.

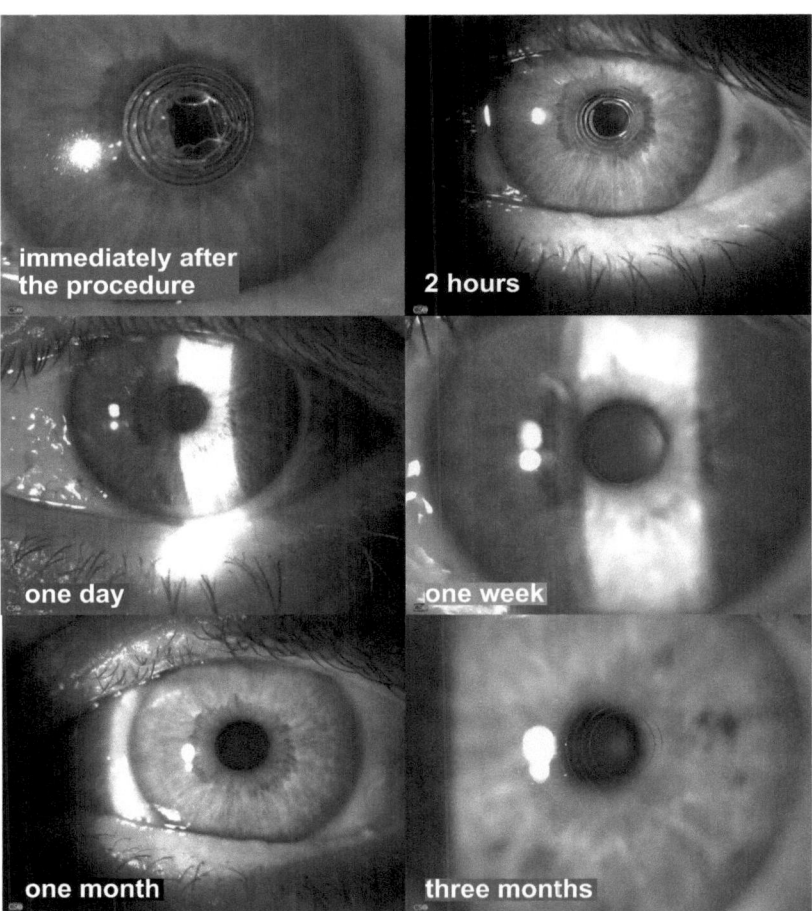

Figure 6.1: Slit-lamp findings in a presbyopic patient that was treated with INTRACOR, immediately after the procedure, 2 hours, one day, one week, one month and three months postoperatively.

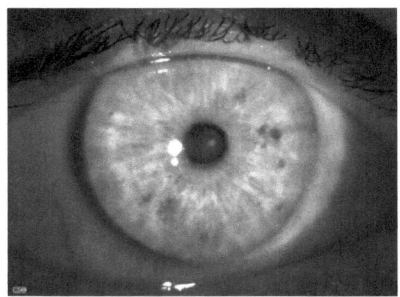

Figure 6.2: The same eye as in figure 6.1. six months postoperatively. The ring cuts can now barely be seen.

3 months postoperatively the mean SE was 0.01±0.46 (range -0.75 to +0.75D). There was statistically significant difference in comparison to pre-operative findings (p=0.003). Mean monocular UDVA was 0.87±0.13 (range 0.7 to 1.0) which was significant as compared to preoperative results (p=0.04) (Figure 6.4). Furthermore, mean monocular UNVA was 0.89±0.18 (range J1 to J16), which was statistically significant in comparison to preoperative values (p=0.004)(Figure 6.5). Mean binocular UDVA was 0.94±0.06 and mean binocular UNVA was 0.90±0.19 (range J1 to J16).

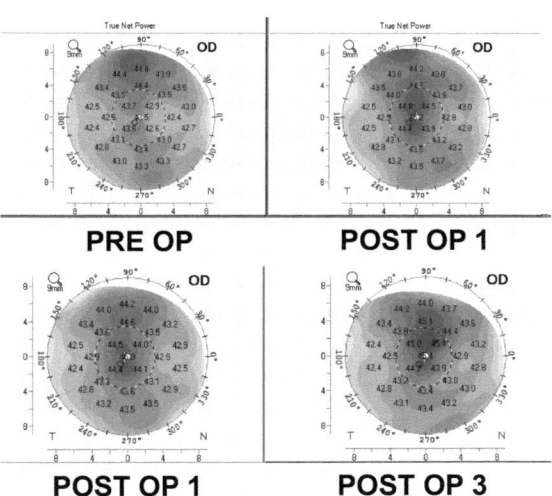

Figure 6.3: Comparison of preoperative with postoperative topography of eye treated with INTRACOR procedure one week, one month and 3 months postoperatively.

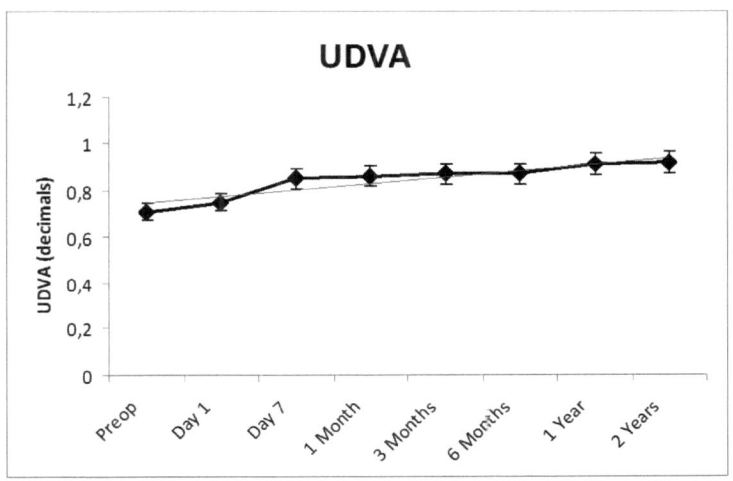

Figure 6.4: Mean monocular uncorrected distance visual acuity UDVA over time.

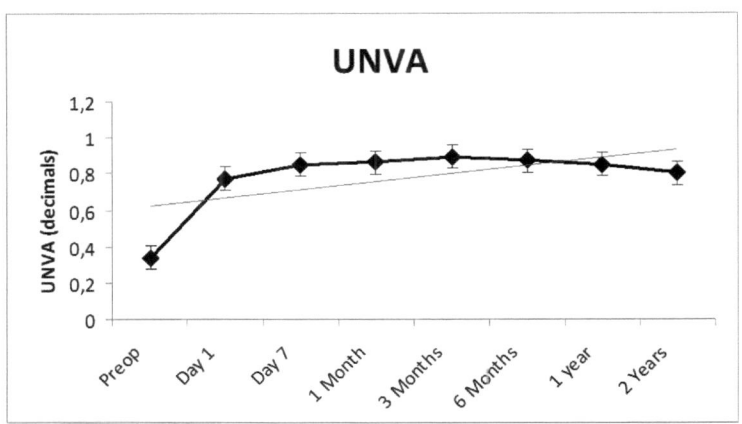

Figure 6.5: Mean monocular uncorrected near visual acuity UNVA over time.

There was no difference in the results between 3 and 6 months postoperatively (p=1.0), and results remained stable over the first postoperative year (p=0.90). However, at the two years follow up slight improvement in monocular distance visual acuity and decrease in monocular near visual acuity were observed. There was no change in patients' binocular visual performances.

At two years follow up mean monocular UDVA was 0.92±0.08 (range 0.7 to 1.0), however there was no statistically significant difference in comparison to 1 year results (p=0.26). Also, mean monocular UNVA was 0.8±0.24 (range J1 to J16) which was not statistically significant as compared to 1 year results (p=0,34).

Postoperative median central steepening increased by 1,8D (range from -0.2 to 2.7D) and remained almost unchanged during postoperative period (p=1,0). There were no correlation between central corneal steepening and gain in UNVA. There was no change in corneal pachymetry before and after the treatment or during the follow up (preoperative 550±30µm, postoperative 546±43µm) (p=0.75). None of the patients developed corneal ectasia or any other corneal irregularity during the whole postoperative period.

The most disturbing side effect was dry eye. Insufficient quality of the tear film caused decrease in near and distance vision quality and increase in night vision disturbances. However, symptoms resolved from few weeks up to few months on frequent administration of the artificial tears.

Overall patients' satisfaction was very good. In the first few weeks after the surgery some patients had mild night vision disturbances such as halo and glare. Night vision disturbances disappeared in all patients from few weeks up to six months after the surgery. Most of the patients noticed dependence of near vision quality on light conditions. In dim light conditions reading ability decreased up to 4 lines and 40% of patients did use some reading glasses for small print in low light conditions. 10% of patients (mostly emmetropic ones) did have complaints about the decreased quality of distance vision in a first few weeks after the surgery. However, after some time they adopted to a new condition and in their opinion quality of distance vision in operated eye increased to a satisfying level.

7 | Overview of literature

**Marija Anticic MD,
Natasa Draca MD,
Nikica Gabric MD, PhD**

Overview of literature
Marija Anticic MD, Natasa Draca MD, Nikica Gabric MD, PhD

Multiple studies have demonstrated that treatment of presbyopia, using a femtosecond laser (INTRACOR), is safe and predictable surgical procedure with stability of visual and corneal outcomes. Nevertheless, as any kind of procedure, it has advantages and disadvantages.

Patients treated with INTRACOR procedure showed significant improvement in uncorrected near visual acuity (UNVA) which occured within some minutes up to a few hours after the treatment and was stable for up to 2 years in most of the cases. Two years after surgery, all eyes gained UNVA which improved from 0,34±0,2 to 0,8±0,24 (median range J16 to J1). Results from other authors had similar median UNVA improvement from J13 to J3. Median gain of UNVA was 4,67 lines (range from 2,5-6) and no eye lost a line of CDVA during a two year period. According to some studies, median gain in UNVA was 4 lines and 3,4% eyes achieved a gain of 9 lines.[1] Other studies showed similar results with gain of UNVA, which ranged from 0 to 9 lines, with stability of results during the one year follow up.[2,3] It remains unclear why certain patients show only a slight gain in near vision.[4]

The fact that some eyes gained only one to three lines indicates a certain number of „low responders". So far, no factors, such as preoperative keratometry, corneal thickness as well as a ring centration have been found to have an impact on the predictability of the postoperative refractive results.[1]

Median CNVA was J1 before and two years after surgery in all patients. Median uncorrected distance visual acuity (UDVA) improved from 0.71±0.21 to 0,87±0,13 (range 0,7 to 1,0) 3 months postoperatively. No difference was noted in UDVA 1 year after surgery, while at two years follow up mean UDVA showed slight improvement and was 0,92±0,08. However, a mild decrease in UDVA from 0.95 to 0.8, due to minimal myopic shift, was observed in 22,2% of patients, 3 months postoperatively. Other studies showed median UDVA of 0,80 before and 1 year after surgery, while some observed a slight decrease in

UDVA from 0,80 to 0,6 18 months postoperatively.[1,2]

Improvement as well as decrease in UDVA could be explained due to myopic refraction shift, and it depends, among all, on the preoperative refraction. As most of the patients were slight hyperopes before the procedure, myopic shift brought their refraction closer to zero and UDVA improved.

In our study median CDVA remained stable for all eyes and was 0,98±0,03 preoperatively, and 0,97±0,04 postoperatively. In some other studies CDVA decreased, which can be very disturbing for patient. Holzer et al. reported 7,1 % of patients who lost two lines of CDVA.[1] Other studies reported 15 % of patients who lost two lines of CDVA.[4] A slight decrease in CDVA could be related to quality of vision due to a change in the depth of focus induced by the treatment, and perhaps by changes in contrast sensitivity.

Postoperative median central steepening increased by 1,8D (range from 0.0 to 2.7D) after two years and remained statistically unchanged (p=1,0, Student's t-test) during postoperative period without any signs of further steepening or corneal ectasia induced by this procedure. Our results are similar with other studies, which reported increase in postoperative median central steepening from 1.05D to 1.40D after 12 months.[2,4]

Some authors have reported corneal steepening of 0,1D after 1 month and -0,1D after 18 months. Despite of the low corneal steepening, this patient gained 5 lines of UNVA.[2]

This fact indicates that low level of corneal steepening in the visual axis does not automatically induce a lack of gain in UNVA. Some other factors could be involved, such as changes in the spherical aberration or corneal asphericity.

We did not measure the change in pre-and postoperative median anterior corneal asphericity. According to Holzer et al change in pre- and postop (12 months) median anterior corneal asphericity was statistically significant and turned toward negative values.[1]

There were no significant changes in pachymetry at the thinnest point over two years (p=0.08) which was similar with other studies.[2]

Contrast sensitivity (CS) was not examined in our study. Some authors reported slight decrease in mesopic contrast sensitivity and increase in glare sensitivity. Results showed that 36 % of patients had decrease in CS without glare, while 52% had decrease in CS with glare.[5]

Knorz et al showed that 90% of patients could see rings around the light while driving at night. These rings are nothing like those induced by a multifocal IOLs and patients have minimal complaints. In fact these rings typically disappear between 6 weeks to 3 months postoperatively However, possible consequences on the night driving ability should be discussed with the patients prior to the treatment.[6]

In our study none of the patients developed cataract after INTRACOR procedure during the 2 years of follow up. In cataract surgery after INTRACOR procedure, as described in case report by Fitting A et al, intraocular lens power calculation is reliable and no adaptation of formulas are needed.[7]

We can conclude that INTRACOR treatment has an effect on improvement of UNVA. However, treatment is still to some extent unpredictable since there are some patients also described as low responders which do not benefit from the procedure. The problem is unreliable preoperative identification of these patients since there is still no known cause for this failure. INTRACOR procedure is limited to the treatment of slightly hyperopic patients because of known postoperative myopic shift of approximately-0,50D.

Future aspects that need to be investigated are different INTRACOR patterns to correct low degrees of myopia and astigmatism. Further long term investigations are needed on large groups of patients to evaluate the feasibility and the outcomes of patients retreatment.

References:

1. Holzer MF, Knorz MC, Tomalla M, Neuhann TM. Intrastromal Femtosecond Laser Presbyopia Correction: 1-year Results of a Multicenter study. J Refract Surg. 2012;28:182-188.

2. Menassa N, Fitting A, Auffhart GU, Holzer MP. Visual outcomes and corneal changes after intrastromal femtosecond laser correction of presbyopia. J Cataract Refract Surg. 2012; 38:765-773.

3. Holzer MP, Mannsfeld A, Ehmar A, Auffarth GU. Early outcomes of INTRACOR femtosecond laser treatment for presbyopia. J Refract Surg. 2012; 28; 182-188.

4. Thomas BC, Fitting A, Auffarth GU, Holzer MP. Femtosecond Laser Correction of presbyopia (INTRACOR) in Emmetropes Using a Modified Pattern. J. Refract Surg. 2012; 28:872-878.

5. Fitting A, Menassa N, Auffhart GU, Holzer MP. Effect of intrastromal correction of presbyopia with femtosecond laser (INTRACOR) on mesopic contrast sensitivity. Ophtalmologe 2012; 109:1001-1007.

6. Knorz MC, 12-Month Conformite Europeenne Data on INTRACOR; Supplement to Cataract and Refractive Surgery Today Europe June 2010.

7. Fitting A, Rabsilber TM, Auffhart GU, Holzer MP. Cataract surgery after previous femtosecond laser intrastromal presbyopia treatment. J Cataract Refract Surg. 2012;38:1293-1297.

Abbreviations

INTRACOR - intrastromal femtosecond laser correction of presbyopia

IOL - intraocular lens

SEB - scleral expansion bands

PMMA - polymethylmethacrylate

CK - conductive keratoplasty

LTK - yttrium–aluminium–garnet laser thermal keratoplasty

UDVA - uncorrected distance visual acuity

CDVA - corrected distance visual acuity

UNVA - uncorrected near visual acuity

CNVA - corrected near visual acuity

LASIK - Laser-Assisted in situ Keratomileusis

CE - Conformite Europeenne

D - diopter

SE - spherical equivalent

µm - micrometer

J - Jaeger score for near visual acuity

CS - Contrast sensitivity

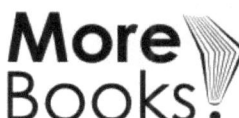
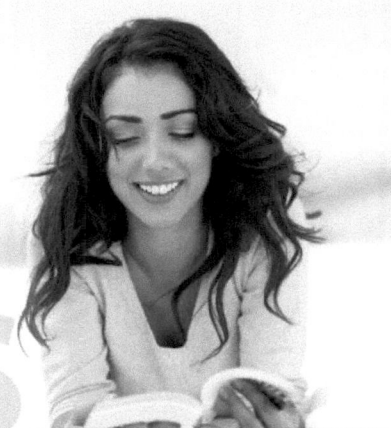

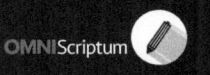

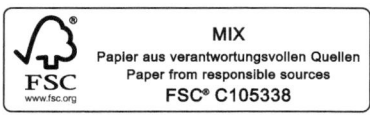